The Book of Everything: vol. 1

Self Discovery

The Book of Everything: vol. 1
Self Discovery

by
Whitley Charee

Copyright © 2018 by BlackGold Publishing
All rights reserved. No part of this book may be reproduced, scanned, or distributed in any printed or electronic form without permission. First Edition: December 2018
Printed in the United States of America
ISBN: **978-0-9995106-6-7**

"Healing is not linear."
I love you. Eddie.

Self Discovery

Self Discovery is described in the dictionary as the process of acquiring insight into one's own character. Simply put, this means learning what it is that makes you tic. Likes, dislikes, passions and everything in between. Most people feel lost and misguided, searching for answers in books, friends and even celebrity idols. Trying to discover what should be important to them. While all this searching actually yields no real results, they fail to look to the one person that actually does hold the answers. Themselves. We have all heard the saying, the truth shall set you free. While this statement is true it doesn't come without weight. The motivation behind this book was a break up. (how cliché, I know) I was in this relationship for seven long years! We met in high school and started dating in college. The relationship moved pretty quickly considering my young age and little real experience in this particular area. Nonetheless I fell in love, tossed most of my friends aside and moved in with my beau. By the age of twenty I was so engulfed in this person I would have done anything to keep them happy, even if at my expense. The funny thing is, they were the exact same way. Everything I wanted, I pretty much got. Sound perfect, huh? Well, not exactly. This actually became the beginning of a pretty codependent emotional roller coaster. Before we knew it our sole existence became as one, we were a unit and everything was OURS. She shared likes, she shared hobbies. We didn't do anything apart, we shared every facet of our lives with each other. It was like we didn't have separate identities. It didn't take long for that to begin to feel pretty claustrophobic for someone like me. (a person with self-identity issues, commitment issues, and d; all of the above) The more serious our relationship got, the more conflicted I began to feel. Who am I? What do I want? What are my values? I had everything everyone would have wanted, but still incredibly unhappy. I did everything under the sun to self-sabotage (drinking, making everyone a priority, but her) Not to say she wasn't also at fault for her own things, but I'm accepting ownership of my shortcomings, only. The things I can control are tied only to me. Anyways, we broke up because my destructive behavior (among many other things, but again self-accountability). It caused a lot of shit and the relationship just couldn't handle the stress of the constant betrayal. So, I left. Upon leaving, I was filled with confusion and didn't even know what I enjoyed doing for fun. Pretty Pathetic. So, I was somewhat forced into self-discovery. I was forced to rediscover myself, be alone in my thoughts and really tune in on why I was the way I was. These same concepts, the ones in this book are tools I had to use. I had to become transparent and force myself to look in the mirror. Considering I didn't like what was looking back, I knew it was time to change the reflection — We tend to hide ourselves from ourselves, especially the ugly parts. I'm here to tell you, those are some of the most important lessons. Part of standing in your truth is going deep. DEEP in the trenches. Typically, where you've stored your traumas, shame, guilt, fears, rejections, shameful actions, pretentious tendencies, and then deciding to free yourself from the baggage. Part of that is understanding the effects of them and why it yielded certain decisions. Understanding that your response to these things are all a part of your make up, but also a mark of continuation for growth and enlightenment. As you continue to navigate through life and move forward to be the best decent human, use whatever has affected you to make you better. Ugliness and All. This book has been designed to meet you where you are and help you in discovering what is important to you, what you need to overcome and resources to ensure your journey continues to prosper long after completing this. This process of self-discovery is never ending, however, this Book of Everything will surely give you the tools needed to continue to grow in your truth. Happy writing.

With Love,

Whitley Charee

Self Care Tip Number 1:

Be Patient With Yourself— It's no coincidence that this is number one. Throughout this journey you will open some wounds, learn new things about yourself (both good and bad) and you will notice a lot of things you want to change about yourself and your thinking. Take it one day at a time. When you feel yourself get off track, gently redirect your thinking so that you find your way back. Don't punish yourself for your slip-ups. For instance, when practicing gratitude, you will have days where gratitude is the furthest from your mind. You will be frustrated about how your life is working out and that okay! That's normal and we all go through it. This book won't erase the problems in your life, but certainly help you deal with them head on. Taking away the power and giving you the ability to focus on things you can actually control.

> "No matter how hard reality seems;
> Just hold onto your dreams."
>
> —Optimistic x Sounds of Blackness

"GOOD THINGS TAKE TIME."

Writing Prompts:

This section will ask you the important questions that will help you sort out all your thoughts.

Some will feel very easy while others feel rather gut wrenching to answer. Be patient with yourself, but also be very transparent. The more honest are the more likely you will actually take something remarkable away. I challenge you to leave everything in the pages, your tears, your fears, your insecurities because it's those very things that will spark your growth.

I am the happiest when...
(What are things that truly make me feel joy)

What am I most afraid of?
(Dig deep and not only identify what your fears are, but also are they rational? Why are you so afraid of this particular thing?)

How can I become proud of the person I am today?
(What changes can you make to be the best version of yourself? What are things that you would like to see yourself possess?)

Whitley Charee's – The Book of Everything, vol 1

What is one thing I've always thought but was too afraid to actually say? Why have I been hiding it?
(It can be anything, small or big. Is there an idea you've been holding onto, an opinion?)

**Am I living my life to the fullest potential or am I product of my past?
If a product of my past, what past experiences am I holding onto?**
(If you are holding onto past experiences, why is that experience so significant to you? What is the takeaway?)

What are my values?

(In this section, be sure to identify the difference between bad/good values. Make sure they are open-ended. Example: Instead of getting married or starting a family, a healthy value would be practicing healthy relationships because by doing that your chances of the above are more likely and won't stop once you obtain those things. Other examples; honesty, respect, compassion.)

I feel anxiety when...
(What are things that make you feel uneasy? Why do you get so anxious in these moments?)

Is my current environment enriching me or depleting me?
(Are people and situations around you giving you energy or draining you?)

If I could change one thing about myself or my life, what would it be?
(I know most of us would want to say nothing, surprise, but try and be transparent in this section. What do you want to change? What do you think those changes will benefit?)

Whitley Charee's – The Book of Everything, vol 1

If I had to write a letter to my past self what would it say?
(I left this open on purpose. I don't care what age self you write to. Based on the age you choose *sometimes* that means you have a significant event that may have been unresolved.)

Am I taking anything for granted?
How can I better practice gratitude?

(This topic gets overlooked a lot, but is very necessary in personal growth. Think about that quote; "Gratitude unlocks the fullness of life" Think about what that means to you.)

Am I spending a lot of time stressing over things I cannot control?
(When you spend time stressing over things out of your control it turns into anxiety. What are things you stress over, again like fear, are they rational? Are they things in your control?)

Am I living a life that is true to myself? If not, why?

(This prompt is so necessary. A lot of times we are living a life that our parents want, our friends want and if you aren't living the life you truly desire this can cause resentment. What are things you truly want and are too afraid to act on? Are things things in your control? Can you make them happen?)

Am I taking care of myself physically?
If not, what changes can I make?
(Mental health is more than the mind, it is feeding the mind good things. The food you eat, the music you listen to and the activities you engage in? How are you treating yourself all around?)

Am I achieving goals that I am setting for myself? If not, why?
(What are some goals I've set for myself in the past? Have a achieved them? What stopped you from reaching this goal or goals?)

Self Care Tip Number 2:

Accept Yourself Above All Else — This can be a rather difficult one. Accepting what you see in the mirror is so important. That includes your short-comings. Accepting yourself at all stages of your process with make the growth even better. By accepting yourself, flaws and all it allows you love yourself without condition. see, if you choose to only love the good qualities of yourself you will get frustrated with yourself when you aren't becoming who you desire fast enough. You want to love yourself as you build yourself. It's okay to acknowledge you are a work in progress and still growing, but don't let the things you are still working on stop you from appreciating how far you have already come in your journey.

"Breathe in and let it go.
Your tears are not for nothing."

—Something Beautiful x Tori Kelly

love yourself

Whitley Charee's – The Book of Everything, vol 1

If no one was around to judge you, what is the one thing you would do?
(Dig deep— What do you look like when no one is watching?)

What makes you feel completely alone?
(What or who is it that makes you feel alone even in a room full of people?)

What is the one thing about myself that frustrates me?
(What are things about myself that I would like to change?)

When is the last time I laughed so hard my stomach began to hurt?
(Think of a time that generated so much laughter that you couldn't contain it. Why is this moment so memorable?)

Where is it that you feel complete and utter peace?
(If I can't think of locations think of factors that aid in feeling peace.)

What am I recovering from right now?
(Is there something that is really heavy on my heart currently?)

What is the last thing I experienced that truly inspired me?
(Can be something I saw, read, or heard)

What do I need right now?
(Think of anything you need in the moment or phase of life?)

What makes you stand out among other people?
(What do I find special about myself?)

What are the traits I look for in a good friend?
(This question is very important because sometimes we settle for people that are generally good, but not always good for ourselves. Be personal with myself. What does a good friend look like to me?)

What is my favorite way to spend a lazy day?
(No work and no obligations, how are you spending the day?)

What song am I connecting with right now? And why?
(Is there a current song I have on repeat? Why is this song so significant?)

Do I enjoy going out or staying inside?
(This one can change frequently so be sure to check in. What do I desire— going out with a group of people, maybe alone or do I prefer to stay in?)

Write about a time where you lost track of time.
(Has something ever had my attention to the point that I lost track of time?)

Is there an ex I would consider dating again? If so, what made them so special? If not, what made them a point of no return?
(Exes are always fun to talk to about— LOL)

_____
_____
_____
_____
_____
_____
_____
_____
_____
_____
_____
_____
_____
_____
_____
_____
_____
_____
_____
_____
_____
_____
_____
_____
_____
_____

What does emotional availability mean to you? Are you emotionally available or emotionally unavailable? Explain—
(Being able to define these things will help you decipher where you are on your journey. No right or wrong. What does this mean to me?)

Whitley Charee's – The Book of Everything, vol 1

What is something that made me angry recently? How did I respond? Why did I get so angry?
(Don't only access what makes us upset, but also how we respond.)

Describe little things in life that make life worth living?

(India Arie mentions the little things best. Just as she believes, I believe the little things to have the most significance. What little things grab my attention and tug at my heart?)

Who is someone you look up to? What about them makes you idolize them?

(This can be anyone, young or old. Famous or familiar. Why is this person so significant? What about them makes you aspire to be more like them?)

What does self-care look like to you?
(What is it going to take for me to divulge in self-love? What am I placing importance on during this journey?)

Have I gone through a break up recently? What did it feel like? Was it my fault? What could I have done differently? What did you need from them?
(Break up aren't only defined by romantic partners? Have a friend and I fallen out? Did I go through a dramatic change in my life? Have a lost someone important to me at all?)

If I could start a business right now what would it be? What would it consist of? Who are my consumers? Is this something I can actually do?

(A lot of us have desires of having our own businesses, Let's start the brainstorming)

Is there someone you are constantly trying to appease? What would you do if you didn't care what they thought?
(Am I giving the power of my life to someone else? Do I make decisions based on what they might think or feel?)

What is the most annoying/frustrating thing a person can do?

(Identifying these things about yourself help you dissolve bad relationships around you. What annoys me? What are my pet peeves? Why does it bother me so much?)

Whitley Charee's – The Book of Everything, vol 1

What is my favorite thing about myself?
(This can be physical, but I challenge you to refer to characteristics. Quality traits make up feel better about ourselves.)

What is the most selfless thing you have ever done for another person?

(Have you ever done anything for another person despite how it would affect me? Have I ever made a decision that would ultimately hurt me to make sure someone was else was happy?)

Whitley Charee's – The Book of Everything, vol 1

Self Care Tip Number 3:

Be Selfish— This on some people may disagree with you, but being selfish is very needed in this journey. When I say be selfish, I mean be selfish with your time, your energy. Be selfish with your entire being. Truth is; everyone doesn't deserve you your time, your frustrations and your energy. Learn to decide what's important. Learn to say no when you don't want to do something. Learn how to create that "me" time for yourself. Learn to focus on things that fuel your spirit and not diminish it. Choose yourself, every time.

"Living life on my time, even if it takes too long."

—Lost x Faarrow

ME
Me
me

Weekly Plans/Goals

This section will help you set goals and actually, accomplish them. They say when you write down a goal the chances of you achieving that goal tremendously improves. I want you to think of any and all goals; personal goals, life goals and career goals. This may seem like an easy task, but thinking about the things you have discovered about yourself this part is pertinent to the overall growth process. Now that you are beginning to see the areas of improvement in your life, this is the time to set realistic goals to better your living experience. Now everything won't occur immediately, but you will notice the changes taking place, you will hold yourself accountable and then a new being will begin to emerge.

Goal:
_____
_____

Why Is this goal important to you?
_____
_____
_____
_____

Is this a long-term goal or short-term goal? (Circle One)
Is this goal realistic? Why or Why not?
_____
_____
_____

What is your deadline on this goal?
_____
_____

What are the steps to accomplishing this goal?
1._____
_____

2._____
_____

3._____
_____

4._____
_____

5._____
_____

COMPLETE THIS PORTION **AFTER** GOAL HAS BEEN MET

Did you meet your deadline? Yes or No? (Circle One)
How did accomplishing this goal make you feel?

Goal:
_____
_____

Why Is this goal important to you?
_____
_____
_____
_____

Is this a long-term goal or short-term goal? (Circle One)
Is this goal realistic? Why or Why not?
_____
_____
_____

What is your deadline on this goal?
_____
_____

What are the steps to accomplishing this goal?
1._____
_____

2._____
_____

3._____
_____

4._____
_____

5._____
_____

COMPLETE THIS PORTION **AFTER** GOAL HAS BEEN MET

Did you meet your deadline? Yes or No? (Circle One)
How did accomplishing this goal make you feel?

_____
_____
_____
_____
_____
_____
_____
_____
_____
_____
_____
_____
_____
_____
_____
_____
_____
_____
_____
_____
_____
_____
_____
_____
_____
_____
_____
_____
_____
_____
_____
_____
_____
_____
_____

Goal:
_____
_____

Why Is this goal important to you?
_____
_____
_____
_____

Is this a long-term goal or short-term goal? (Circle One)
Is this goal realistic? Why or Why not?
_____
_____
_____
_____

What is your deadline on this goal?
_____
_____

What are the steps to accomplishing this goal?
1._____
_____

2._____
_____

3._____
_____

4._____
_____

5._____
_____

Whitley Charee's – The Book of Everything, vol 1

COMPLETE THIS PORTION **AFTER** GOAL HAS BEEN MET

Did you meet your deadline? Yes or No? (Circle One)
How did accomplishing this goal make you feel?
_____
_____
_____
_____
_____
_____
_____
_____
_____
_____
_____
_____
_____
_____
_____
_____
_____
_____
_____
_____
_____
_____
_____
_____
_____
_____
_____
_____
_____
_____
_____
_____
_____
_____
_____
_____

Goal:
_____
_____

Why Is this goal important to you?
_____
_____
_____
_____

Is this a long-term goal or short-term goal? (Circle One)
Is this goal realistic? Why or Why not?
_____
_____
_____

What is your deadline on this goal?
_____
_____

What are the steps to accomplishing this goal?
1._____
_____
_____

2._____
_____
_____

3._____
_____
_____

4._____
_____
_____

5._____
_____
_____

COMPLETE THIS PORTION **AFTER** GOAL HAS BEEN MET

Did you meet your deadline? Yes or No? (Circle One)
How did accomplishing this goal make you feel?
_____
_____
_____
_____
_____
_____
_____
_____
_____
_____
_____
_____
_____
_____
_____
_____
_____
_____
_____
_____
_____
_____
_____
_____
_____
_____
_____
_____
_____
_____
_____
_____
_____

Goal:
_____
_____

Why Is this goal important to you?
_____
_____
_____
_____

Is this a long-term goal or short-term goal? (Circle One)
Is this goal realistic? Why or Why not?
_____
_____
_____

What is your deadline on this goal?
_____
_____

What are the steps to accomplishing this goal?
1._____
_____

2._____
_____

3._____
_____

4._____
_____

5._____
_____

Whitley Charee's – The Book of Everything, vol 1

COMPLETE THIS PORTION **AFTER** GOAL HAS BEEN MET

Did you meet your deadline? Yes or No? (Circle One)
How did accomplishing this goal make you feel?

Goal:
_____
_____

Why Is this goal important to you?
_____
_____
_____
_____

Is this a long-term goal or short-term goal? (Circle One)
Is this goal realistic? Why or Why not?
_____
_____
_____
_____

What is your deadline on this goal?
_____
_____

What are the steps to accomplishing this goal?
1._____
_____

2._____
_____

3._____
_____

4._____
_____

5._____
_____

COMPLETE THIS PORTION **AFTER** GOAL HAS BEEN MET

Did you meet your deadline? Yes or No? (Circle One)
How did accomplishing this goal make you feel?

_____
_____
_____
_____
_____
_____
_____
_____
_____
_____
_____
_____
_____
_____
_____
_____
_____
_____
_____
_____
_____
_____
_____
_____
_____
_____
_____
_____
_____
_____

Goal:
_____
_____

Why Is this goal important to you?
_____
_____
_____
_____

Is this a long-term goal or short-term goal? (Circle One)
Is this goal realistic? Why or Why not?
_____
_____
_____
_____

What is your deadline on this goal?
_____
_____

What are the steps to accomplishing this goal?
1._____
_____

2._____
_____

3._____
_____

4._____
_____

5._____
_____

Whitley Charee's – The Book of Everything, vol 1

COMPLETE THIS PORTION **AFTER** GOAL HAS BEEN MET

Did you meet your deadline? Yes or No? (Circle One)
How did accomplishing this goal make you feel?

_____
_____
_____
_____
_____
_____
_____
_____
_____
_____
_____
_____
_____
_____
_____
_____
_____
_____
_____
_____
_____
_____
_____
_____
_____
_____
_____
_____
_____
_____
_____
_____

Goal:
_____
_____

Why Is this goal important to you?
_____
_____
_____
_____

Is this a long-term goal or short-term goal? (Circle One)
Is this goal realistic? Why or Why not?
_____
_____
_____
_____

What is your deadline on this goal?
_____
_____

What are the steps to accomplishing this goal?
1._____
_____

2._____
_____

3._____
_____

4._____
_____

5._____
_____

Whitley Charee's – The Book of Everything, vol 1

COMPLETE THIS PORTION **AFTER** GOAL HAS BEEN MET

Did you meet your deadline? Yes or No? (Circle One)
How did accomplishing this goal make you feel?

_____
_____
_____
_____
_____
_____
_____
_____
_____
_____
_____
_____
_____
_____
_____
_____
_____
_____
_____
_____
_____
_____
_____
_____
_____
_____
_____
_____
_____

Goal:
_____
_____

Why Is this goal important to you?
_____
_____
_____
_____

Is this a long-term goal or short-term goal? (Circle One)
Is this goal realistic? Why or Why not?
_____
_____
_____
_____

What is your deadline on this goal?
_____
_____

What are the steps to accomplishing this goal?
1._____
_____
_____

2._____
_____
_____

3._____
_____
_____

4._____
_____

5._____
_____
_____

Whitley Charee's – The Book of Everything, vol 1

COMPLETE THIS PORTION **AFTER** GOAL HAS BEEN MET

Did you meet your deadline? Yes or No? (Circle One)
How did accomplishing this goal make you feel?

Goal:
_____
_____

Why Is this goal important to you?
_____
_____
_____
_____

Is this a long-term goal or short-term goal? (Circle One)
Is this goal realistic? Why or Why not?
_____
_____
_____

What is your deadline on this goal?
_____
_____

What are the steps to accomplishing this goal?
1._____
_____

2._____
_____

3._____
_____

4._____
_____

5._____
_____

COMPLETE THIS PORTION **AFTER** GOAL HAS BEEN MET

Did you meet your deadline? Yes or No? (Circle One)
How did accomplishing this goal make you feel?

_____
_____
_____
_____
_____
_____
_____
_____
_____
_____
_____
_____
_____
_____
_____
_____
_____
_____
_____
_____
_____
_____
_____
_____
_____
_____
_____
_____
_____
_____
_____
_____
_____
_____

Goal:
_____
_____

Why Is this goal important to you?
_____
_____
_____
_____

Is this a long-term goal or short-term goal? (Circle One)
Is this goal realistic? Why or Why not?
_____
_____
_____
_____

What is your deadline on this goal?
_____
_____

What are the steps to accomplishing this goal?
1._____
_____

2._____
_____

3._____
_____

4._____
_____

5._____
_____

COMPLETE THIS PORTION **AFTER** GOAL HAS BEEN MET

Did you meet your deadline? Yes or No? (Circle One)
How did accomplishing this goal make you feel?

Goal:
_____
_____

Why Is this goal important to you?
_____
_____
_____
_____

Is this a long-term goal or short-term goal? (Circle One)
Is this goal realistic? Why or Why not?
_____
_____
_____
_____

What is your deadline on this goal?
_____
_____

What are the steps to accomplishing this goal?
1._____
_____

2._____
_____

3._____
_____

4._____
_____

5._____
_____

COMPLETE THIS PORTION **AFTER** GOAL HAS BEEN MET

Did you meet your deadline? Yes or No? (Circle One)
How did accomplishing this goal make you feel?
_____
_____
_____
_____
_____
_____
_____
_____
_____
_____
_____
_____
_____
_____
_____
_____
_____
_____
_____
_____
_____
_____
_____
_____
_____
_____
_____
_____
_____
_____
_____
_____
_____
_____
_____
_____

Goal:
_____
_____

Why Is this goal important to you?
_____
_____
_____
_____

Is this a long-term goal or short-term goal? (Circle One)
Is this goal realistic? Why or Why not?
_____
_____
_____

What is your deadline on this goal?
_____
_____

What are the steps to accomplishing this goal?
1._____
_____

2._____
_____

3._____
_____

4._____
_____

5._____
_____

COMPLETE THIS PORTION **AFTER** GOAL HAS BEEN MET

Did you meet your deadline? Yes or No? (Circle One)
How did accomplishing this goal make you feel?

Goal:
_____
_____

Why Is this goal important to you?
_____
_____
_____
_____

Is this a long-term goal or short-term goal? (Circle One)
Is this goal realistic? Why or Why not?
_____
_____
_____

What is your deadline on this goal?
_____
_____

What are the steps to accomplishing this goal?
1._____
_____

2._____
_____

3._____
_____

4._____
_____

5._____
_____

Whitley Charee's – The Book of Everything, vol 1

COMPLETE THIS PORTION **AFTER** GOAL HAS BEEN MET

Did you meet your deadline? Yes or No? (Circle One)
How did accomplishing this goal make you feel?

_____
_____
_____
_____
_____
_____
_____
_____
_____
_____
_____
_____
_____
_____
_____
_____
_____
_____
_____
_____
_____
_____
_____
_____
_____
_____
_____
_____
_____
_____
_____
_____
_____

Goal:
_____
_____

Why Is this goal important to you?
_____
_____
_____
_____

Is this a long-term goal or short-term goal? (Circle One)
Is this goal realistic? Why or Why not?
_____
_____
_____
_____

What is your deadline on this goal?
_____
_____

What are the steps to accomplishing this goal?
1. _____
_____

2. _____
_____

3. _____
_____

4. _____
_____

5. _____
_____

Whitley Charee's – The Book of Everything, vol 1

COMPLETE THIS PORTION **AFTER** GOAL HAS BEEN MET

Did you meet your deadline? Yes or No? (Circle One)
How did accomplishing this goal make you feel?

_____
_____
_____
_____
_____
_____
_____
_____
_____
_____
_____
_____
_____
_____
_____
_____
_____
_____
_____
_____
_____
_____
_____
_____
_____
_____
_____
_____
_____
_____
_____
_____
_____
_____
_____
_____
_____

Goal:
_____
_____

Why Is this goal important to you?
_____
_____
_____
_____

Is this a long-term goal or short-term goal? (Circle One)
Is this goal realistic? Why or Why not?
_____
_____
_____
_____

What is your deadline on this goal?
_____
_____

What are the steps to accomplishing this goal?
1._____
_____

2._____
_____

3._____
_____

4._____
_____

5._____
_____

COMPLETE THIS PORTION **AFTER** GOAL HAS BEEN MET

Did you meet your deadline? Yes or No? (Circle One)
How did accomplishing this goal make you feel?

Goal:
_____
_____

Why Is this goal important to you?
_____
_____
_____
_____

Is this a long-term goal or short-term goal? (Circle One)
Is this goal realistic? Why or Why not?
_____
_____
_____
_____

What is your deadline on this goal?
_____
_____

What are the steps to accomplishing this goal?
1._____
_____
_____

2._____
_____
_____

3._____
_____
_____

4._____
_____
_____

5._____
_____
_____

Whitley Charee's – The Book of Everything, vol 1

COMPLETE THIS PORTION **AFTER** GOAL HAS BEEN MET

Did you meet your deadline? Yes or No? (Circle One)
How did accomplishing this goal make you feel?

_____
_____
_____
_____
_____
_____
_____
_____
_____
_____
_____
_____
_____
_____
_____
_____
_____
_____
_____
_____
_____
_____
_____
_____
_____
_____
_____
_____
_____
_____
_____
_____
_____
_____

Goal:
_____
_____

Why Is this goal important to you?
_____
_____
_____
_____

Is this a long-term goal or short-term goal? (Circle One)
Is this goal realistic? Why or Why not?
_____
_____
_____
_____

What is your deadline on this goal?
_____
_____

What are the steps to accomplishing this goal?
1._____
_____

2._____
_____

3._____
_____

4._____
_____

5._____
_____

Whitley Charee's – The Book of Everything, vol 1

COMPLETE THIS PORTION **AFTER** GOAL HAS BEEN MET

Did you meet your deadline? Yes or No? (Circle One)
How did accomplishing this goal make you feel?

_____
_____
_____
_____
_____
_____
_____
_____
_____
_____
_____
_____
_____
_____
_____
_____
_____
_____
_____
_____
_____
_____
_____
_____
_____
_____
_____
_____
_____
_____

Goal:
_____
_____

Why Is this goal important to you?
_____
_____
_____
_____

Is this a long-term goal or short-term goal? (Circle One)
Is this goal realistic? Why or Why not?
_____
_____
_____
_____

What is your deadline on this goal?
_____
_____

What are the steps to accomplishing this goal?
1._____
_____

2._____
_____

3._____
_____

4._____
_____

5._____
_____

COMPLETE THIS PORTION **AFTER** GOAL HAS BEEN MET

Did you meet your deadline? Yes or No? (Circle One)
How did accomplishing this goal make you feel?
_____
_____
_____
_____
_____
_____
_____
_____
_____
_____
_____
_____
_____
_____
_____
_____
_____
_____
_____
_____
_____
_____
_____
_____
_____
_____
_____
_____
_____
_____
_____
_____
_____
_____
_____

Goal:
_____
_____

Why Is this goal important to you?
_____
_____
_____
_____

Is this a long-term goal or short-term goal? (Circle One)
Is this goal realistic? Why or Why not?
_____
_____
_____
_____

What is your deadline on this goal?
_____
_____

What are the steps to accomplishing this goal?
1._____
_____

2._____
_____

3._____
_____

4._____
_____

5._____
_____

COMPLETE THIS PORTION **AFTER** GOAL HAS BEEN MET

Did you meet your deadline? Yes or No? (Circle One)
How did accomplishing this goal make you feel?
_____
_____
_____
_____
_____
_____
_____
_____
_____
_____
_____
_____
_____
_____
_____
_____
_____
_____
_____
_____
_____
_____
_____
_____
_____
_____
_____
_____
_____
_____
_____
_____

Whitley Charee's – The Book of Everything, vol 1

Self Care Tip Number 4:

Control What You Can Control— Our biggest downfall sometimes is stressing over things we can't control. When we let these things take up our mental space, we find ourselves feeling helpless. You begin to feel exhausted because you are constantly anxious over things you can't change. Instead, I want you to look at things in your life that you can change. What are things that are causing you to be unhappy that you can actually change? Once you shift the direction of your thinking you will begin to feel more in control of your mental space and your life as a whole.

"One Step at a time. There's no need to rush; It's gon happen when it's supposed to happen."

—One Step at A Time x Jordin Sparks

NOTE TO SELF:
relax

Free Space

This section is the space to just have your way! If you are a writer, journal. If you are a musician, write a few lines to a song. If you like to draw, doodle away! This section is dedicated to you and all of you. If you feel the urge to jot down some feelings or if you just want to draw a simple picture, this is the area to do it! There are no rules, no limitations, JUST YOU! Explore that creative space and let it run wild. You'd be amazed at the things you'd come up with when you silence your mind.

Yes, (in case you're wondering) the following pages are left **intentionally blank!**

Go on, ENJOY!

Whitley Charee's – The Book of Everything, vol 1

Whitley Charee's – The Book of Everything, vol 1

Whitley Charee's – The Book of Everything, vol 1

Self Care Tip Number 5:

Declutter the Spaces Around You— This one is small, but you'd be surprised the difference this makes. Clean your bedroom, light some candles, stop hanging out with people that make you feel about bad about yourself. Get rid of anything that doesn't serve a positive purpose in your life. I promise it's really that simple. I always hear more season adults say, "A cluttered space leads to a cluttered mind." Clear the space around you and watch it make you feel better.

"It's okay not to be okay"

— Who You Are x Jessie J

tidy desk tidy mind

More Free Space –
With lines this time for journaling, of course!

More Free Space –
With lines this time for journaling, of course!

**More Free Space –
With lines this time for journaling, of course!**

More Free Space –
With lines this time for journaling, of course!

More Free Space –
With lines this time for journaling, of course!

More Free Space –
With lines this time for journaling, of course!

Whitley Charee's – The Book of Everything, vol 1

More Free Space –
With lines this time for journaling, of course!

More Free Space –
With lines this time for journaling, of course!

Whitley Charee's – The Book of Everything, vol 1

**More Free Space –
With lines this time for journaling, of course!**

More Free Space –
With lines this time for journaling, of course!

Whitley Charee's – The Book of Everything, vol 1

More Free Space –
With lines this time for journaling, of course!

More Free Space –
With lines this time for journaling, of course!

More Free Space –
With lines this time for journaling, of course!

More Free Space –
With lines this time for journaling, of course!

Whitley Charee's – The Book of Everything, vol 1

More Free Space –
With lines this time for journaling, of course!

More Free Space –
With lines this time for journaling, of course!

More Free Space –
With lines this time for journaling, of course!

More Free Space –
With lines this time for journaling, of course!

More Free Space –
With lines this time for journaling, of course!

More Free Space –
With lines this time for journaling, of course!

Whitley Charee's – The Book of Everything, vol 1

**More Free Space –
With lines this time for journaling, of course!**

Self Care Tip Number 6:

Set Boundaries with Yourself and Others — This one gets over looked a lot in the self-exploration process. Setting boundaries is important because you want to make it clear to yourself and others what you want and don't want. If you want to be alone, say that. If you want that job, apply for it. If you wanna ask that guy out, do it. Exist with intention. Create your boundaries and follow through.

> "I'm alone, but I'm not lonely. Comfortably indulging and trying to get to know me."
>
> —Confidently Lost x Sabrina Claudio

the secret to getting ahead is getting started

Conclusion

Congratulations!

You did it and I am incredibly proud. It's not always easy sitting down with yourself and putting in the necessary work to heal and better yourself, but you did it. This is only the beginning. The journey of self-discovery and personal reflection never actually ends. It's an ongoing process. I am glad that you chose to utilize my resource to help you along the way!

I hope that you walk into your journey more self-aware, more open to try new things, readily accepting of yourself and others. But most of all, I hope you walk into your journey truly loving yourself. No one Is perfect, we are only human and sometimes we are the hardest on ourselves. Today starts a new day for you— be gentle with yourself, speak life into your spirit, be patient if you don't see changes right away (because most likely you won't) This is a chance for you to really get into yourself and connect. We connect with family, friends, co-workers, so why is it so easy to neglect connecting with ourselves. I poured my all into this book and I really hope that it serves you how it has served me this past year! These resources should and will continue to offer you the support on your personal journey. Just because you are finished with the pages doesn't mean you are finished evolving. I want to see you continue to journey!

Peace, love and vibrations,
Xoxo
Whitley Charee

Letter to my supporters:

Over the past year I have undergone tremendous changes; From moving out of my old apartment, leaving a long-term relationship, loosing friends and starting a new job. You guys have been nothing short of amazing. You continuously encourage and uplift me so I have the strength to produce artistic and creative material. I've haven't been producing much during this past year because it was necessary for me to step back and reflect on all the changes happening. During this time, you all gave me love, understanding and patience.

I couldn't ask for better supporters in my corner.

I hope that you enjoyed this as much as I did creating it.

I wanted to show that this time away has not been in vain and that I am still growing even behind closed doors I love each and every one of you. You've calmed my tears, you've picked me up on the bad days, you've given me perspective on things when I was upset. The only thing that hasn't changed is, I work hard for YALL! IF I make it, we all win!

Thanks for the support,
I love you
Whitley C Dickson

"We were in so deep. We could barely thread, but now I found a way to heal myself instead."

—Alive x Kehlani